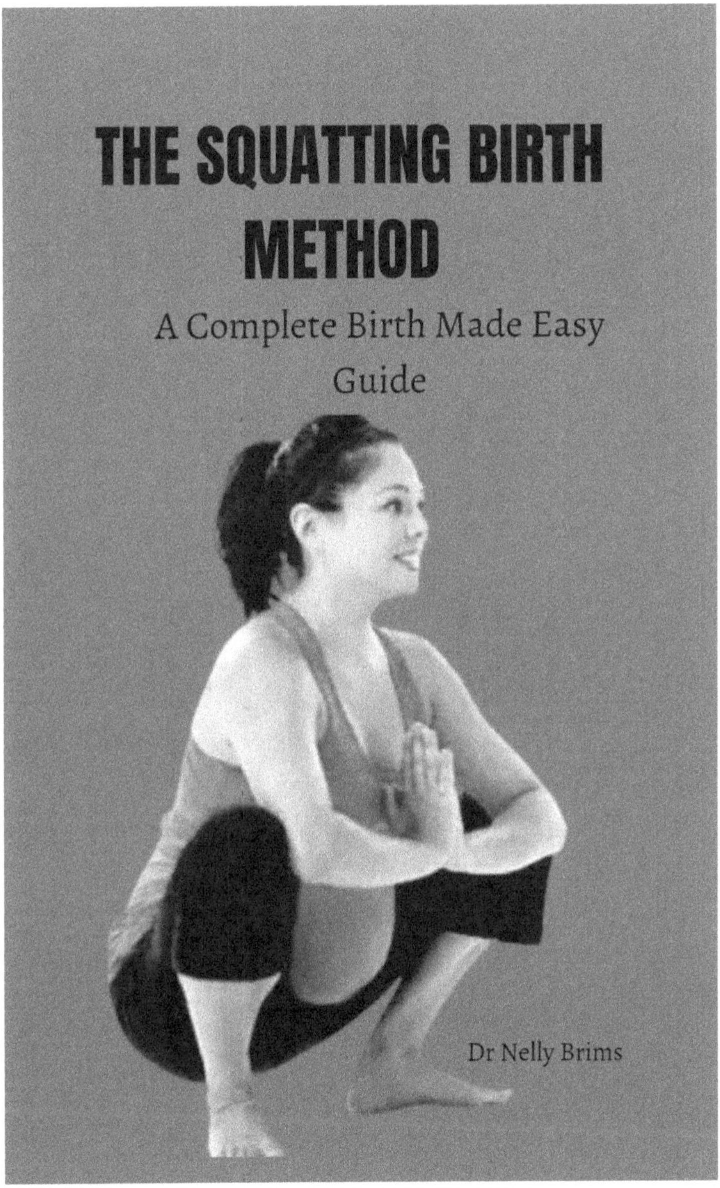

THE SQUATTING BIRTH METHOD

A Complete Birth Made Easy Guide

Dr Nelly Brims

THE SQUATTING BIRTH METHOD

A COMPLETE BIRTH MADE EASY GUIDE

By Dr Nelly Brims

TABLE OF CONTENTS

INTRODUCTION

Notwithstanding many years of examination, the occasions prompting the commencement of work in people stay hazy. It is thought that biochemical substances delivered by the baby initiate work. Likewise, the planning of the development of these substances and their cooperation with placental and maternal biochemical variables seem to impact this interaction. Among the most contemplated of these biochemical substances are fetal chemicals like oxytocin and placental provocative particles. Expanded placental and maternal creation of fiery atoms in late pregnancy has been emphatically connected to the commencement of work. Hormonelike substances called prostaglandins, which are delivered by the placenta in light of different biochemical signs, can prompt aggravation and are available in expanded levels during work. A few factors that increment the development of prostaglandins incorporate oxytocin, which invigorates the power and recurrence of uterine withdrawals, and a fetal lung protein considered surfactant protein A (SP-A). Surfactant creation in the fetal lung doesn't start until the last phases of growth, when the hatchling plans for air breathing; this change might go about as a significant work switch.

The phases of work
First stage: dilatation

Right off the bat in labor, uterine compressions, or work torments, happen at time frames to 30 minutes and last around 40 seconds. They are then joined by slight agony, which generally is felt in the little of the back.

As work advances, those withdrawals become more extraordinary and dynamically expand in recurrence until, toward the finish of the primary stage, when dilatation is finished, they repeat about like clockwork and are very extreme. With every compression a twofold impact is created to work with the dilatation, or opening, of the cervix. Since the uterus is a strong organ containing a liquid filled sac called the amnion (or "pack of waters") that pretty much encompasses the youngster, constriction of the muscle structure of its walls ought to decrease its pit and pack its items. Since its items are very incompressible, nonetheless, they are constrained toward least opposition, which is toward the isthmus, or upper opening of the neck of the uterus, and are driven, similar to a wedge, increasingly far into this opening. As well as driving the uterine items toward the cervix, shortening of the muscle strands that are appended to the neck of the uterus will in general draw those tissues up and away from the opening and subsequently adds to its broadening. By this consolidated activity every withdrawal of the uterus not just powers the amnion and hatchling lower against the widening neck of the uterus yet additionally pulls the opposing walls of the last option vertically over the propelling amnion, introducing part of the youngster.

Britannica Test Going to Pop: What number of Children? Disregarding this apparently viable component, the term of the principal phase of work is somewhat delayed, particularly in ladies who are in the process of giving birth interestingly. In such ladies the typical time expected for the finish of the phase of dilatation is somewhere in the range of 13 and 14 hours, while in ladies who have recently brought forth kids the normal is 8 to 9 hours. Besides the fact that a past work will in general abbreviate this stage, however the propensity frequently increases with succeeding pregnancies, with the outcome that a lady who has brought forth three or four kids might have a first phase of one hour or less in her next work.

The principal phase of work is remarkably drawn out in ladies who become pregnant interestingly after age 35, in light of the fact that the cervix expands less promptly. A comparative deferral is to be expected in cases in which the cervix is broadly scarred because of past works, removal, profound burning, or some other surgery on the cervix. Indeed, even a lady who has borne a few kids and whose cervix, as needs be, ought to expand promptly may have a drawn out first stage assuming the uterine compressions are frail and rare or on the other hand in the event that the kid lies in a badly designed position for conveyance and, as an immediate result, can't be constrained into the mother's pelvis.

Get a Britannica Premium membership and get sufficiently close to selective substance.

Buy in At this point
Then again, the early cracking of the amnion frequently
expands the strength and recurrence of the work
torments and subsequently abbreviates the phase of
dilatation; once in a while, untimely loss of the amniotic
liquid prompts embellishment of the uterus about the
youngster and in this way defers dilatation by
forestalling the kid's typical plunge into the pelvis.
Similarly as a strange place of the youngster and trim of
the uterus might forestall the typical plunge of the kid, an
unusually huge kid or an unusually little pelvis might
impede the plummet of the kid and draw out the main
phase of work.

Second stage: ejection
About the time that the cervix turns out to be completely
enlarged, the amnion breaks, and the power of the
compulsory uterine withdrawals might be increased by
intentional pushing ahead endeavors of the mother. With
each work torment, she can take a full breath and
afterward contract her muscular strength. The expanded
intra-stomach pressure subsequently created may rise
to or surpass the power of the uterine withdrawals.
These pushing ahead endeavors might twofold the
viability of the uterine compressions.

As the kid drops into and goes through the birth trench,
the vibe of agony is frequently expanded. This condition
is particularly obvious in the terminal period of the phase
of removal, when the youngster's head stretches and
widens the maternal tissues as it is being conceived.

Fetal show and entry through the birth waterway
Consecutive changes in the place of the kid during work.
How the kid goes through the birth waterway in the
second phase of work relies on the situation in which it
is lying and the state of the mother's pelvis. The
grouping of occasions depicted in the accompanying
passages is what much of the time happens when the
mother's pelvis is of the typical kind and the kid is lying
with the highest point of its head lowermost and
dynamically positioned and the rear of its head (occiput)
coordinated toward the left half of the mother (see
beginning of work in the figure). The highest point of the
head, likewise, is driving, and its long hub lies
transitionally.

The power received from the uterine withdrawals and
the pushing ahead endeavors applies strain on the
youngster's bottom and is sent along the vertebral
section to drive the head into and through the pelvis. On
account of the connection of the spine to the foundation
of the skull, the rear of the head propels more quickly
than the forehead with the outcome that the head
becomes flexed (i.e., the neck is bowed) until the jaw
comes to lie against the breastbone (see flexion in the
figure). As an outcome of this flexion instrument, the
highest point of the head turns into the main post and
the ovoid head boundary that entered the birth waterway
is prevailed by a more modest, practically round
periphery, the long width of which is around 2 cm (0.75
inch) more limited than that of the prior outline.

As the head plummets all the more profoundly into the birth channel, it meets the obstruction of the hard pelvis and of the slinglike pelvic floor, or stomach, which slants descending, forward, and internal. At the point when the rear of the head, the main piece of the youngster, is constrained against this slanting wall on the left side, it normally is shunted forward and to the right as it progresses (see interior turn of head in the figure). This inner revolution of the head carries its longest breadth into connection with the longest width of the pelvic outlet and subsequently enormously aids the variation of the propelling head to the arrangement of the cavity through which it is to pass.

Further drop of the head straightforwardly descending toward the path where it has been voyaging is gone against by the lower piece of the mother's hard pelvis, behind, and the opposing delicate parts that are mediated among it and the launch of the vagina (see interior pivot of head in the figure). Less opposition, then again, is presented by the delicate and dilatable walls of the lower birth trench, which is coordinated forward and up. The rear of the kid's head as needed be propelled along the lower birth waterway, distending its walls and expanding its depression while the head advances. Before long the rear of the kid's neck becomes encroached against the bones of the pelvis, and the jawline is constrained increasingly far away from the breastbone. Consequently, as expansion (bowing of the head in reverse) replaces flexion, the occiput, temple, eye attachments, nose, mouth, and jawline go progressively through the outer opening of the lower birth waterway and are conceived (see augmentation in the figure).

The neck, which was bent during the inside turn of the head, untwists when the head is conceived. Very quickly after its introduction to the world, accordingly, the highest point of the head is moved in the direction of the left and in reverse.

As the youngster's lower shoulder progresses, it meets the slanting opposition of the pelvic floor on the right side and is shunted forward and to the left close to the center of the pelvis in front. This position brings the long measurement of the shoulder perimeter into connection with the anteroposterior, or long distance across, of the pelvic cavity. In view of this inside pivot of the shoulders, the highest point of the head goes through additional outside revolution in reverse and to the left so the kid's face comes to gaze straight toward the inward part of the mother's right thigh (see outer turn of head in the figure).

Not long after the shoulders pivot, the one in front shows up in the vulvovaginal hole and stays here while the other shoulder is cleared forward by a sidelong bowing of the storage compartment through the very up and advance bend that was trailed by the head as it was being conceived. After this shoulder is conveyed, experienced in 3 to 4 percent of conveyances. Since the head in such cases is the last piece of the kid to be conveyed and on the grounds that this piece of the conveyance is the most troublesome, the umbilical string might be packed while the aftercoming head is being conceived, with the outcome that the kid might be suffocated. Asphyxia or wounds to the kid that result from the chaperon's work to rush the conveyance to forestall the youngster's suffocation are liable for the deficiency of three fold the number of breech infants as head-on children. Consequently the kid might be maneuvered toward a head-on position by the specialist or be conveyed by the surgery called cesarean segment.

The baby death rate in created nations changes from 2 to 10 percent as per the size of the youngster and ability of the chaperon. Since tiny untimely newborn children are especially helpless to the risks of breech conveyance, the mortality among them is exceptionally high when they are conceived first.

Britannica Test Going to Pop: What number of Infants?
Crossover show
In this somewhat uncommon circumstance the long pivot of the youngster will in general lie across, or cross over to, the long hub of the mother. Except if the youngster is tiny, conveyance through the regular entries is unimaginable in such cases; thus, conveyance by cesarean segment is vital.

Since the previously mentioned complexities are rare and can be really focused on effectively, the maternal demise rate is under 1 for every 1,000 and would be still lower assuming the passings brought about by confounding fundamental infections were rejected. The newborn child death rate is likewise low, running somewhere in the range of 1.5 and 3 percent. It would be a lot lower in the event that untimely and ineffectively created newborn children were rejected. At the end of the day, the gamble to a solid mother who conveys her youngster to development is under 1 for each 1,000, and the gamble to her full grown kid is around 0.5 percent.

Third stage: placental stage
With the ejection of the kid, the hole of the uterus is extraordinarily decreased (see uterus following birth in the figure). As an outcome, the site of placental connection turns out to be notably decreased in size, with the outcome that the placenta (fetal membrane) is isolated in many spots from the layer covering the uterus. Inside a couple of moments resulting uterine withdrawals complete the division and power the placenta into the vagina, from which it is removed by a pushing ahead exertion. The third phase of work, in like manner, is of brief length, rarely enduring longer than 15 minutes. Sporadically, be that as it may, the partition might be deferred and joined by dying, in which case careful evacuation of the placenta is vital.

Alfred C. Beck

Alleviation of agony in labor
Torment experienced in labor can be decreased or eased by psychoprophylaxis, fundamental medications, territorial nerve blocks, or a mix of those techniques. Perhaps the earliest medication to be utilized for help with discomfort was chloroform, which was at first utilized in the last part of the 1840s yet ultimately came into neglect on account of its harmfulness. In the mid twentieth century a combination of scopolamine, an amnesic medication, and morphine was given to deliver "nightfall rest." On arousing from the prompted fanciful express, the lady would have no memory of her work torments. The longing to be a functioning member in the birth insight and to keep away from the results of ridiculousness and pipedreams prompted surrender of this methodology.

Since originally portrayed during the 1930s, psychoprophylaxis has acquired ubiquity as a strategy for mentally and truly setting up a person for labor, in this way assisting her with expecting and adapting to the aggravation of work (see underneath Normal labor). What's more, an agreeable and lovely climate, strong loved ones, and an equipped and empowering birth chaperon can assist with lessening or even kill the requirement for drug relief from discomfort. Nobody's strategy, nonetheless, is fit to each lady. Medications and methods that are at present being used are portrayed momentarily in the accompanying segments.

Foundational drugs

Meperidine and morphine, given intravenously, are normal opiate drugs utilized for help with discomfort (absence of pain) during work. There are secondary effects related with the two medications — to be specific, queasiness and regurgitating. At the point when promethazine is given related to meperidine, these incidental effects are improved. Other negative maternal impacts brought about by foundational analgesics are tiredness, respiratory melancholy, and bringing down of circulatory strain (hypotension). Since fundamental medications cross the placental boundary, they can likewise influence the infant, causing respiratory gloom, diminished readiness, and unusual reflexes. The more drawn out the span between the organization of the opiate and the introduction of the youngster, the higher the level of the medication in the baby and the more noteworthy its belongings. One more medication regularly utilized for fundamental absence of pain is butorphanol, which delivers less neonatal misery.

Barbiturates, once significant for diminishing work torments, are currently just seldom controlled during work. Despite the fact that they are tranquilizers, which regularly prompt a casual state, they are not analgesics and really may expand aversion to torment. Barbiturates additionally cause respiratory sadness in the infant assuming directed in dynamic work, which can be exacerbated by the associative utilization of opiate analgesics. Tranquilizers are utilized exclusively in the beginning phases of work to help the lady unwind and rest before the compressions of dynamic work start.

Neighborhood sedation

Worries about the adverse consequences that foundational medications might have on the mother and infant have prompted weighty dependence on nearby sedation. Nearby sedative specialists work by forestalling the conduction of nerve driving forces. Their activities are restricted to sensory tissue situated close to the infusion site, due to their capacity to diffuse just brief distances. In this manner, neighborhood sedatives numb just a confined piece of the body and permit the lady to hold cognizance, clarity, and command over the remainder of her body.

Epidural block

The lumbar epidural block has become one of the most famous options for the executives of work torment in the US. The most well-known sedatives utilized are bupivacaine and lidocaine. At the point when a catheter is utilized, the upsides of this strategy incorporate the capacity to change portion, volume, and sort of sedative, as suitable to the phase of work. In the event that a cesarean conveyance becomes vital, the epidural sedation can be reached out to give relief from discomfort to the technique. Issues related with a lumbar epidural block incorporate bringing down of maternal circulatory strain and urinary maintenance. Since this system can slow work, the chemical oxytocin is frequently regulated simultaneously to animate uterine constrictions.

Spinal sedation

Spinal sedation (some of the time called spinal block) is created when a nearby sedative specialist, like lidocaine or bupivacaine, once in a while blended in with an opiate, is infused into the cerebrospinal liquid in the lumbar district of the spine. This strategy permits the lady to be alert, while delivering broad desensitization of the mid-region, legs, and feet. Since it is a solitary infusion, its length is restricted, by and large going on around two hours, contingent upon the portion. Therefore, spinal sedation is regularly held for cesarean areas or is managed during work when conveyance is normal in two hours or less. A sort of spinal sedation called a seat block anesthetizes the inward thighs, hindquarters, and perineum — the pieces of the body that in a sitting position would come into contact with a seat. The desensitizing impact once in a while stretches out past the expected seat region, notwithstanding, coming to the extent that the toes. Outrageous maternal hypotension, a diminishing in utero-placental perfusion, and loss of the desire to push are taking a chance that can go with spinal sedation. These impacts, as well as the notoriety of more normal labor encounters and of epidural block, added to a decrease in the utilization of this strategy.

Pudendal block

The pudendal block is a moderately straightforward and normal technique that numbs the birth waterway and perineum for unconstrained conveyance, forceps conveyance, vacuum extraction, and episiotomy. Similar sedative specialists utilized in epidural sedation are utilized and are infused through the vagina to the pudendal nerve. This method alleviates the aggravation from perineal distension however not from uterine compressions.

Normal labor
During the 1930s Grantly Dick-Read, an English obstetrician, fostered a method of conveyance called normal labor that limited the careful and sedative parts of conveyance and concentrated upon the mother's cognizant work to bring forth her youngster. Albeit went against by numerous doctors who felt that it denied the advancement of current medication and unnecessarily primitivism the course of birth, the technique was step by step acknowledged and by the last part of the 1950s was rehearsed by a sizable level of ladies, particularly in the US and Britain.

Normal labor — in some cases called psychoprophylaxis, arranged labor, or the Lamaze strategy — as figured out by Dick-Read and later high level by Fernand Lamaze, Elisabeth Bing, Robert Bradley, and Charles Leboyer, comes from the reason that labor need not be joined by exorbitant agony. It is accepted that work torments are the consequence of unnatural actual strain brought about by dread, which can be neutralized by understanding and by fostering the capacity to unwind. The different strategies recommend for the eager mother and an accomplice an extensive course of guidance in the mechanics of work and birth as well as activities to reinforce the muscle structure and to empower legitimate relaxation. Accentuation is put on including other relatives, particularly the dad, in the birth cycle. During her work the mother is supported via prepared staff and her accomplice, or "mentor," and sedatives are made accessible to her when required.

heaviness or discomfort in the pelvic cavity, and difficulty in emptying the lower bowel. The bulging mass formed by a cystourethrocele (protrusion of the bladder and urethra into the vagina) or rectocele (protrusion of the rectum into the vagina), found during a pelvic examination, confirms the diagnosis. Uterine prolapse may be so severe that the uterus lies completely outside the vagina, and the vagina is turned inside out. Treatment depends on the severity of the symptoms; severe prolapse is repaired surgically.

Inversion of the uterus
Another complication that may occur during labor is inversion of the uterus. The uterus turns inside out and upside down so that its inner surface lies outside and against the wall of the vagina. Inversion causes sudden hypotension and shock, and there may be severe bleeding. The diagnosis is made by noting the uterus, covered by a dark red, bleeding surface, filling or protruding outside the vagina. The placenta may be attached to the uterus.
The Editors of Reference book Britannica
Employable obstetrics

Most ladies convey a child precipitously.
Notwithstanding, confusions that were available before
work or that create during work might undermine the
existence of the mother or of the child and may require
mediation by the going to doctor.

Cesarean area

At the point when a kid can't be conveyed through the
vagina, it very well might be important to fall back on
cesarean segment, a technique in which the embryo is
conveyed through a careful opening made in the uterus
after the uterus has been uncovered through an opening
made in the stomach wall. The cesarean segment
developed from being a surgery utilized exclusively in
outrageous cases and from which the mother seldom
recuperated to perhaps of the most usually carried out
strategy in the US. Before the twentieth 100 years,
ladies going through a cesarean segment normally
created peritonitis and passed on. Not until the coming
of aseptic procedure, trustworthy sedation, and
legitimate stitching strategies that controlled drain was
the cesarean conveyance thought about a sensible
option in contrast to vaginal conveyance.

Cesarean conveyance is viewed as fitting in different
circumstances in which the dangers of vaginal
conveyance to the embryo or mother are considered to
be more prominent than the dangers from stomach
conveyance. Normal signs for the method incorporate
disappointment of work to advance, unexpected labor
for clinical reasons, fetal pain, and ill-advised situating of

the baby for conveyance. Furthermore, cesarean segment is frequently utilized assuming the birth trench is excessively little for vaginal conveyance. The method is utilized to stay away from additional drain when there is draining from placenta praevia (connection of the placenta to the uterine wall so that it covers the cervix) or from a rashly isolated placenta. On the off chance that the mother is contaminated with repetitive genital herpes and injuries are clear at the hour of conveyance, a cesarean conveyance is normally suggested. It is likewise dependent on the event that a lady's circulatory strain rises sharply during work, as can happen with toxemia (albeit, by and large, vaginal conveyance is desirable over cesarean conveyance for ladies with toxemia). Uncommon cases, for example, an oddity of the genitalia or a crippled solid issue that keeps the mother from pushing during work, will by and large require this methodology.

Maternal complexities are as yet connected with the cesarean segment. Blood misfortune, injury to the inside or bladder, and contamination are normal dangers. Recuperating of the entry point additionally protracts recuperation. Although the system is much of the time accomplished to serve the baby in danger from asphyxia or injury coming about because of a vaginal birth, there are related neonatal dangers. Newborn children who have been conveyed at different gestational ages once in a while foster respiratory disease. The reason isn't totally perceived, however the disorder is most frequently found in babies conveyed centrally without any work. Incidental slashes of the baby with the surgical tool in some cases happen. Cesarean conveyance likewise is connected with a higher frequency of placenta praevia in ongoing pregnancies.

In the late twentieth 100 years there was worry that the cesarean segment, albeit a lifesaving system in circumstances wherein either the lady or the kid could never have endured conveyance in any case, was becoming abused. From the 1970s, obstetricians progressively depended on cesarean birth as an option in contrast to vaginal birth. The four most successive reasons referred to for performing cesarean segments in the US were drawn out work, fetal pain, breech show, and past stomach conveyance. By 2003 about 28 percent of ladies in the US had cesarean conveyances, which was viewed as too high on account of the dangers and complexities that the cesarean area itself is acquainted with. Be that as it may, more secure careful procedures created in the mid 21st century have enormously diminished the dangers customarily connected with this method, however there is a general pattern in the medical services local area to support vaginal conveyance when cesarean segments are excessive.

Forceps conveyance
Obstetrical forceps are utilized in vaginal conveyance to get a handle on the fetal head to remove the baby or pivot it so it is in a good situation for conveyance. Some discussion encompasses the utilization of this

technique, however it is for the most part concurred that it ought to be utilized in circumstances risky to the mother or hatchling that could be feeling better by brief conveyance. In the event that a quick conveyance is wanted to diminish maternal pressure, particularly on the off chance that the lady has coronary illness, intense pneumonic edema, or certain neurological circumstances or on the other hand in the event that weariness or a delayed second phase of work imperil an effective vaginal conveyance, forceps might be utilized. Fetal signs for the utilization of forceps incorporate prolapse of the umbilical line, untimely detachment of the placenta (placentae), and specific unusual fetal pulses. A specific part of the fetal head genuinely should be jutting from the cervix for this method to be ok for the mother and baby. Extensive consideration should be taken to abstain from harming maternal tissues and causing fetal twisting.

Manual turn might be utilized rather than forceps when the fetal head is in an unusual place that makes conveyance troublesome or unthinkable. In completing the method, the obstetrician's hand is embedded into the birth trench, and the fetal head is gone to a better position.

Vacuum extraction
The vacuum extractor is a caplike gadget that is connected by pull to the fetal scalp and is utilized as an option in contrast to conveyance by forceps. This procedure is utilized more oftentimes in Europe than it is

in the US. Cervical and vaginal injury have happened in ladies going through this technique, however it is less extreme and less continuous than that accomplished with forceps conveyance and is the principal benefit of vacuum extraction over forceps conveyance. Conceivable fetal inconveniences incorporate harm to the scalp and intracranial drain.

The Editors of Reference book Britannica
Inconveniences during work
Slashes
Vaginal gashes typically manifest as bountiful draining after conveyance of the child. Not all broad cuts cause dying, be that as it may, and a huge tear in the vaginal wall may not be found until the medical care supplier reviews the vagina after the placenta is conveyed. There is no trouble in diagnosing gashes close to the outside opening of the birth trench, since they are effortlessly seen by the medical services supplier. Indeed, even minor cuts are fixed, in light of the fact that, on the off chance that they are not, granulation tissue might frame in the injuries and postpone mending. Profound gashes require careful remaking of the torn tissues. Broad tears of the perineum (the tissues between the genital organs and the butt) can frequently be tried not to play out an episiotomy — an entry point in the vulvar hole, the outside genital opening — before conveyance of the newborn child's head. Likewise, consideration on the medical care supplier's part to the system of work, manual help with conveyance of the head and shoulders, evasion of too quick conveyance,

conveyance among torments, and the legitimate utilization of the forceps are a portion of the many estimates that assistance to stay away from wounds not exclusively to the perineum yet to every one of the genital tissues.

The cervix, the lower end of the uterus that undertakes into the vagina, is normally examined after the placenta has been conveyed. Shallow tears seem to be a frayed edge on the cufflike cervix. More profound cuts typically cause serious draining preceding or after conveyance of the placenta, and these slashes should be fixed expeditiously. By and large, little cervical slashes are not fixed, since they mend unexpectedly. In any case, further tears are stitched. The administration of broad attacks on the body of the uterus or the wide tendons that help the uterus relies upon the degree of the injury and its area; stomach a medical procedure is some of the time expected to control draining and to fix the uterus. At times hysterectomy — expulsion of the uterus — is fundamental.

Break of the uterus
Break of the uterus might happen suddenly; it could be brought about by injury, or it might happen when a cesarean-segment scar gives way. The old style indications of looming unconstrained break are continuously expanding, steady, extreme torment in the lower part of the mid-region, fretfulness, a climbing temperature, a rising heartbeat rate, and a strained, delicate uterus that doesn't loosen up major areas of

strength for between. At the point when a burst happens, the patient gripes, typically, of outrageous torment and afterward an impression of something tearing or giving way. Uterine withdrawals stop. There is broad inward dying. The child's body can be felt in the mother's mid-region alongside the contracted uterus. Brief conveyance, quite often by cesarean segment, is the treatment of looming crack. The patient is anesthetized to stop uterine withdrawals when the conclusion is made.

Quick stomach medical procedure follows the finding of uterine break. Draining from the torn uterine walls should be halted as instantly as could be expected. The baby is taken out. A hysterectomy is generally performed, in light of the fact that the worn out uterine scar is probably going to crack once more on the off chance that the patient has another term pregnancy, and draining from the torn uterus is challenging to control. Such patients frequently require liberal amounts of bonded blood. Antimicrobials are given, since contamination is, or might be, available.

Uterine prolapse
Uterine prolapse, or a sliding of the uterus from its generally expected position in the pelvic pit, may result from wounds to the pelvic supporting tendons and muscles that happen during work. Normally the conclusion is made months or even years after the fact, when the patient whines of something distancing from

the vagina, compulsory loss of pee while hacking or
chucklin.

Restoration of a uterus to its normal position is
accomplished after the patient's shock and hemorrhage
are treated and she is anesthetized. The obstetrician
inserts a hand into the patient's vagina and lifts up the
uterus. The tension applied to the uterine ligaments by
this procedure usually reinvents the uterus; if this fails,
surgery is necessary.

CHAPTER 1

THE SQUATTING BIRTH METHOD

Throughout recent hundreds of years, in numerous Western nations, emergency clinic based intrapartum care became standard [1,2]. The explanations behind such a change are multifactorial and have been developing over the long haul. Such a model of obstetrics moved the overall view of pregnancy from a physiological to a neurotic condition. It likewise brought about a decline in lady's portability during work. One of the reasons for this diminishing is taking on a lithotomy position, giving better perineal access at whatever point an instrumental conveyance is required [1]. Another explanation is the expanded utilization of epidural absence of pain [2].

A few ladies solicited to take on a non-lithotomy position during the second phase of work. A precise survey and meta-examination assessing any upstanding situation without epidural proposed an unassuming decrease in the length of the subsequent stage, a decrease in mediations (instrumental conveyance and episiotomy), yet an expansion in blood misfortune [3]. These outcomes were not tracked down in another orderly audit and meta-examination of concentrates in ladies with epidural, including the BUMPES preliminary, the bigger randomized preliminary regarding this matter [4,5]. The aftereffects of the preliminaries remembered for the two audits are heterogeneous, potentially as a result of the consideration of different upstanding positions. We center in this audit explicitly around the hunching down position.

The possible benefits of the crouching position incorporate the impacts of gravity [1,3,6], a superior arrangement of the embryo in the birth channel [7], an increment of the pelvic outlet measurement [[8], [9], [10], [11]], and an expansion in the effectiveness of uterine compressions [1]. Then again, it was accounted for that embracing such a position is related with expanded hazard of peroneal neuropathy [12], a deficiency of lady's body equilibrium and lower effectiveness of the pushing endeavors during the second phase of work [17].

Whether these likely advantages and dangers of crouching position during the second phase of work convert into clinically applicable maternal and fetal results is obscure. To resolve this issue, we played out a methodical survey and meta-investigation of the randomized preliminaries assessing the impacts of taking on a hunching down position during the second phase of work.

2 Techniques
2.1 Information sources

We played out an orderly survey of distributions filed in three significant electronic data sets - Cochrane Focal Register of Controlled Preliminaries (Focal), MEDLINE, and Embase. This large number of data sets were looked at from their individual beginning dates to the fourteenth of December 2019. A total portrayal of the pursuit procedure is given in Reference section A. The arrangements of references in the recognized distributions were physically looked at. No fleeting or territorial limitations were applied.

Creators of the distributions were reached and welcomed to partake in a singular member information meta-examination. Be that as it may, none of the creators answered our greeting.

2.2 Qualification measures
The consideration measures were characterized deduced as follows: 1) sorts of studies: randomized preliminary ; 2) kind of members: pregnant ladies during the second phase of work; 3) mediations: independent crouching position contrasted with any prostrate situation during the second phase of work (positions portrayed in subtleties in Addendum B).

Since most of Western grown-ups see it as troublesome and debilitating to crouch heels down, a few investigations proposed a changed crouching position. In this survey, the preliminaries were rejected in the event that the crouching position was changed utilizing a birth seat, a birth pad or the lady was upheld by someone else. In light of the minor change of the position, utilization of a bar to work with crouching was, nonetheless, not considered as prohibition measures for the review.

2.3 Principal results
1) Essential maternal result measure: span of the second phase of work [minutes]; 2) Optional maternal result measures: method of birth [cesarean area, instrumental conveyance (forceps or vacuum-helped conveyance), unconstrained vaginal delivery], torment [Visual Simple Scale], utilization of any absence of pain [non-epidural analgesia], perineal injury [second-degree tear, third-or/and fourth-degree tear, episiotomy], blood misfortune [> 500 mL blood misfortune (mL)]; paraurethral tears; held placenta; shoulder dystocia; 3) Kinds of neonatal results: Apgar score [1-minute Apgar score and 5-minute Apgar score], admission to neonatal emergency unit, demise.

2.4 Information extraction
Two free analysts (FD and DD) scanned titles and edited compositions for distributions that at first met the incorporation rules. The distributions meeting the standards were all chosen for full-text investigation. Errors were settled by conversation. In this way, the analysts autonomously separated the information and finished the recently pre-arranged structure. Information about the executives was performed utilizing audit supervisor programming (RevMan 5) [13].

2.5 Evaluation of hazard of predisposition
Two free commentators (FD and DD) evaluated the gamble of predisposition of each study utilizing the strategy portrayed in the Cochrane Handbook for Methodical Audits of Mediations (adaptation 5.1.0) [14]. The apparatus assesses choice predisposition [random arrangement age; portion concealment], execution inclination [blinding of members and personnel], recognition inclination [blinding of result assessment], wearing down inclination [incomplete result data], and revealing inclination [selective reporting]. For each included distribution, the gamble of the inclination table was delivered, depicting each surveyed variable and its reviewing as low-, moderate-, and high gamble of predisposition (Informative supplement E). If there should be an occurrence of conflict, a third creator (IMM) was counseled.

Data on financing of the included investigations was looked for.

2.6 Evaluation of the nature of proof
The nature of proof was surveyed utilizing the Reviewing of Proposals, Appraisal, Improvement and Assessments (GRADE) programming [15]. The accompanying results for hunching down and recumbent situation during work were thought about: 1) term of the second phase of work; 2) method of birth [cesarean section]; 3) method of birth [instrumental conveyance for example forceps or vacuum extraction]; 4) torment [VAS]; 5) extreme perineal injury

[third-/fourth-degree tear]; 6) blood misfortune [> 500 mL]; and 7) admission to neonatal serious consideration (Supplement F).

2.7 Measurable investigation

For dichotomous results, we determined the gamble proportion with the 95 % certainty span. For persistent results, when the estimation strategy was comparable, we utilized the mean contrast. Measurable heterogeneity was surveyed in each meta-examination utilizing the Tau^2, I^2, and Chi^2 measurements. The gamble of distribution predisposition couldn't be surveyed involving a test for the unevenness of the pipe plot, since there were just seven included preliminaries. We pooled the impacts by a fixed-impacts meta-examination (Shelf Haenszel technique), except if there was huge heterogeneity between preliminaries. Within the sight of heterogeneity ($I2 > 40$ %), we pooled the assessments of the impacts with the irregular impacts model (reverse difference strategy). The measurable meaning of the pooled not entirely settled with Z-test and P-esteem. We reached by email the comparing creators of the included distributions to enhance missing information. None of the exploration bunches answered to our solicitation. To incorporate information from the concentrate by Moraloglu et al., the Apgar score medians were considered as means and the standard deviation was assessed as half of the reach between the base and the middle 18. Measurable investigation was performed utilizing RevMan 5 [13].

2.8 PROSPERO enrollment number

CRD42018093244

3 Outcomes

3.1 General qualities of the examinations

A sum of 411 distributions were at first distinguished by the information base hunts (Figure A1). Just articles written in English or French were found. In the wake of sifting the titles and modified works, a sum of 14 full-text distributions met the qualification standards [[16], [17], [18], [19], [20], [21], [22], [23], [24], [25], [26], [27], [28], [29]]. At last, after full-text examination, seven randomized controlled preliminaries with a sum of 1219 members were remembered for the quantitative blend (Reference section C) [[16], [17], [18], [19], [20], [21], [22]]. We rejected seven preliminaries since 1) results on crouching position gave other upstanding positions [[23], [24], [25], [26]]; 2) position not relating to the meaning of crouching position [27,28]; 3) prohibition of countless ladies not taking the hunching down position and goal to-treat investigation not revealed 29] (Addendum B and D).

Among the examinations remembered for the quantitative blend, three investigations [17,18,21] included primiparous ladies just, three [16,20,22] concentrates on included both primiparous and multiparous ladies and one review [19] didn't cover equality. A large portion of the investigations' incorporation models were gestational age at 37 weeks or more, with no obstetric or unexpected problems. Lin et al. [17] included members from 38 weeks, and another review didn't give data on gestational age [20]. (Supplement C)

In every one of the included preliminaries, the mediation was characterized as a crouching position, contrasted with the recumbent situation during the second phase of work [[16], [17], [18], [19], [20], [21], [22], [23], [24], [25], [26], [27], [28], [29]]. One review [18] assessed a changed hunching down position, utilizing a bar. Another review [17] broke down both norm and lower leg upheld crouching position, contrasted and prostate. Just the outcomes for the standard crouching position were remembered for the meta-examination.

The examinations were all led in emergency clinics, one in a college emergency clinic [20]. Six of them occurred in AsiaIndia [16], Taiwan [17], Turkey [18], Pakistan [19,22], and Iran [21]) and one in Europe (France [20]). 3 do intercession, including an assortment of crouching positions, time taking the distributed position and utilization of help. We confined the consideration of preliminaries to those assessing crouching position, generally un-supported.

The Terms of the second phase of work were not different between gatherings. The little contrast in the outline gauge was impacted by one review with outrageous outcomes and strangely little standard deviation, which could be because of a normalized convention utilized in this hospital18. The speculation of a decrease in the term of the second phase of work was thought as naturally conceivable as per current information on obstetrical biomechanics. It was accounted for that, in the hunching down position, the pelvic gulf might be nearer to the ideal position [6,30]; there is an expansion in the measurement of the pelvis by around 3% [8,9,31]; the impact of gravity is added to the pushing endeavors [6,10]; there is an expansion in the power of uterine constrictions 1; the place of the embryo in the birth waterway might be improved [17,22]; a superior dissemination of tension on the perineal region builds the desire to push [19,22]; there is a lower hazard of extraordinary vessels pressure and a diminished fetal pressure [18,22,32]. This large number of potential benefits don't, nonetheless, decipher better maternal or neonatal results.

The lower chance of instrumental conveyance might be a certifiable advantage or get from a lower propensity of performing mediations via guardians as a result of restricted perineal access [32,33]. The higher gamble of the cesarean segment in the crouching position is hard to make sense of. This chance is essentially impacted by the aftereffects of one preliminary [22]. The signs were malpresentation (n = 4), postdate pregnancy (n = 2) and toxemia (n = 2), which were avoidance measures. Just 4 cesarean areas were performed for inability to advance. Barring the above circumstances, the gamble of the cesarean segment is lesser and as of now not measurably huge (RR 1.82, 95 %CI 0.75-4.40; 5 preliminaries; 1033 ladies; P = 0.18).

In spite of higher strain applied on the vagina, normal for the hunching down position, the gamble of perineal harm, including third-and fourth-degree tear, was not expanded [34,35]. This might be credited to a more homogeneous dispersion of tensions over the birth trench. Fringe neuropathies, which were raised as a likely worry with hunching down, were not detailed in any preliminary. Blood misfortune and chance of post pregnancy discharge were not expanded in the hunching down position. Just a single report detailed expanded draining in the hunching down position, yet not arriving at the customary limit of 500 mL to characterize discharge [17]. Expanded draining was a worry with other upstanding positions, however this is most likely because of a superior discovery of blood misfortune in these positions, as opposed to a genuine impact.

4.3 Ramifications for clinical practice and field of information

The majority of the included examinations (six out of seven) were directed in Asia, where crouching is regular. Thus, the consequences of this audit might be hard to sum up to Western nations, where the hunching down position is challenging to take on by ladies, who find it awkward and testing to keep up with [17,18,29]. In any case, the consequences of the main European preliminary didn't contrast from Asian examinations, with the exception of lower consistency. In one of the prohibited examinations [29], just 16 % of ladies apportioned to the crouching bunch conceived an offspring here. Embracing a changed crouching position [17], with bars or the help from someone else, may work on the worthiness of the mediation.

4.4 Impediments of the survey
An impediment of the survey is the trouble to normalize the crouching position and to have a uniform span of remaining there. Contrasts between studies might add to the noticed factual heterogeneity.

The modest number of studies and pooled test size, the heterogeneity, the irregularity toward the impact, and the for the most part high or hazy gamble of inclination between included examinations, and the overall low quality of the investigations, demolish the nature of proof and restricts the finishes of this survey. We decide to incorporate just randomized controlled preliminaries, the main review plan that gives a legitimate gauge of the impacts of a mediation. Notwithstanding, there is an absence of providing details regarding the strategies to accomplish randomization and disguise of portions in the vast majority of the examinations.

We couldn't define epidural absence of pain use or equality. It may very well be estimated that outcomes in these sub-gatherings of ladies might not be the same as the general outcomes.

The low quantities of examinations included didn't permit us to distinguish a distribution inclination utilizing a channel plot. There is the chance of such predisposition in this specific circumstance, as little preliminaries not showing a helpful impact may not be distributed in light of the fact that they were against the assessments of that time on the worth of upstanding or crouching position. This is one more constraint of this audit.

5 Ends

In spite of the hypothetical benefits of a crouching position during the second phase of work, this survey shows no helpful or hurtful impact of hunching down during labor. The expansion in cesarean areas is, in any case, concerning. Since there are major areas of strength for not possibly in support of crouching position, ladies ought to be permitted to embrace their preferred place during pushing endeavors, with unbiased directing from the parental figures.

CHAPTER 2

SQUATTING DURING GESTATION

At the point when I previously figured out I was pregnant, I was energized, however with this fervor likewise came interruption. With such countless large changes not too far off, zeroing in on quite a bit of anything was extreme. Whether I was working, shopping for food, or scrubbing down, my brain generally returned to my pregnancy and child.

Unexpectedly, life as far as I might be concerned had such countless contemplations to be made. Might I at any point drink my everyday espresso? What pre-birth nutrients are ideal? Might I at any point actually do my typical exercises?

Fortunately for you, ultimately I had the option to haul my head out of the mists to assemble a few explicit proposals and assets for you moms-to-be considering how and if to change your lifting project to help your body through this section.

The present blog will zero in on Squats during pregnancy as they are one of our #1 activities to integrate into Areas of strength for us programs. Whether you do them with just your body weight, a light hand weight, or a stacked hand weight squats can help you, your child, and work on your work, conveyance, and post pregnancy recuperation!

When you find out you're pregnant, there are countless inquiries, contemplations, stresses, and favors twirling around your brain. In the event that you are a rec center devotee, quite possibly of your greatest concern, the principal will spend several months exploring the exercise center and realizing what practices you can in any case do and how to change them en route.

One of our #1 activities to integrate into Areas of strength for us programs for generally safe moms-to-be are squats. Whether you do them with just your body weight, with a light free weight, or a stacked hand weight, squats can help you, your child, and work on your work, conveyance, and recuperation process!

Numerous maternity specialists and moderate OB's will prescribe hunching down to, as a matter of fact:

Keep up with pelvic floor strength.

Keep your glutes solid, which thus, will balance out your pelvis and diminish lower back torment.

Develop fortitude and perseverance for standing firm on different footings during work and conveyance.

An extra advantage of crouching during pregnancy is to keep up with and additionally assemble muscle in your quads, hamstrings, and glutes for further developed body creation, strength, and metabolic rate during pregnancy and post pregnancy.

What you want to be aware:

In the two or three months of pregnancy you will actually want to hunch down. You generally have absent a lot of progress to position or execution, however you actually need to pay attention to your body. On the off chance that you're feeling depleted or powerless, it's 100 percent alright and suggested that you take the weight, reps, or put it down on a case by case basis. It's likewise time to quit holding back nothing and performing sets or reps where your structure endures by any means.

As your child knock begins developing, your focal point of gravity will change and your hips, back, and inward thighs might feel extra close. As of now, you should be considerably more persistent about doing a legitimate warm-up and you might have to bring the load down more essentially as you conform to changes in your body and to rehearse your new structure.

In general, this weight drop is brief and when you feel more steady in your new influences, you will actually want to build the obstruction piece securely. (Furthermore, in the event that not, that is alright too Mother!)

These are the alterations you might have to make to your squat during pregnancy…

Enlarge your position.

On the off chance that you ordinarily squat with your feet at hip-width, for instance, you will probably have to bring each foot .5-1.5 inches more extensive. This will make more space for your knock to fit between your hips, will give a superior establishment to you to remain adjusted, and will serve to all more uniformly convey your weight.

A more restricted position (in the event that you could in fact get into a full squat like this) will pitch your chest forward and move your hips back which will mess up your bar way, put a burden on your lower back and make a decent morning development design as opposed to a squat.

Uniformly appropriate your breath.

It's normal for experienced lifters to bring their pre-pregnancy diaphragmatic breathing and propping with them into their pregnancy preparation.

The issue with breathing like this is that it can make tension in your stomach by pushing your breath OUT against their linea alba (the line of connective tissue that runs down the center of your stomach). This tension can worsen diastasis recti during pregnancy and past in the post pregnancy period.

You actually need to stomach inhale (IE breath air into stomach, not chest), but rather don't stress such a huge amount over making serious strain and be mindful so as not to simply push out! Equitably convey your breath down, out, up, and back into your lower back.

Stand up against the bar.

Indeed, even with the more extensive position, your new body and influences will make to a greater degree a forward incline in your squat. Rather than considering standing the load up, consider driving once again into the hand weight and wedging your hips forward to escape the opening. (look at shot as an image or video of this)

Slow the unconventional part.

Try not to simply drop into your squat allowing gravity to dominate. Crush the bar, screw your feet in, drive your knees out, and open your… bring down the weight w/control and goal.

Pay attention to your body.

Allow your body to decide the loads you use. It's not an opportunity to be an exercise center class legend. Center around development and meet yourself, and your body, where you're at every day.

Scale when required.

See, you're pregnant. Your body is extending to outrageous lengths to make a human. It's alright to trade out hand weight squats for portable weight squats, leg press, belt squats, box squats or to utilize a light free weight or your bodyweight to take care of business.

You merit a gold star for simply appearing and working out. Try not to be a captive to past achievements. You'll get back there some time or another in the event that you need to.

CHAPTER 3

SQUATTING AND YOUR PELVIS

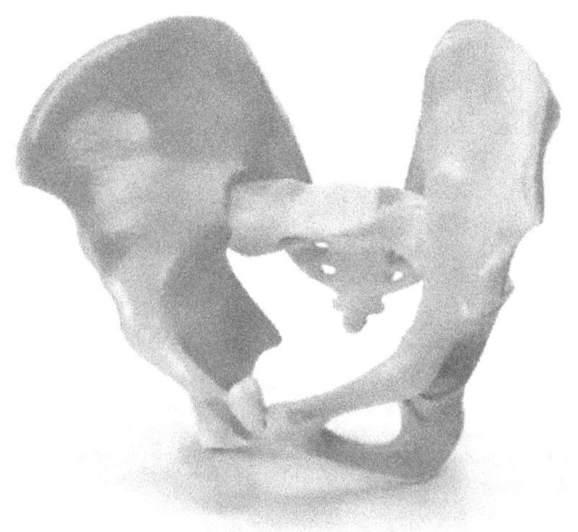

Biomechanical complexities of labor, like impeded work, are a significant reason for maternal and infant bleakness and mortality. The effect of birthing position and portability on pelvic arrangement during work has not been sufficiently investigated. Our goal was to utilize a formerly evolved computational model of the female pelvis to decide the impacts of maternal situating and pregnancy on pelvic arrangement. We conjectured that stacking conditions during crouching and expanded tendon laxity during pregnancy would extend the pelvis. We reproduced dynamic joint minutes experienced during a squat development under pregnant and non-pregnant circumstances while following important physical milestones on the innominate bones, sacrum, and coccyx; anteroposterior and cross over measurements, pubic symphysis width and point, pelvic regions at the gulf, mid-plane, and outlet, were determined. Pregnant reenactment conditions brought about more prominent expansions in most pelvic estimations - and dominatingly at the power source - than for the non-pregnant recreation. Pelvic outlet distances across in front back and cross over headings in the last squat stance expanded by 6.1 mm and 11.0 mm, separately, for the pregnant recreation contrasted and just 4.1 mm and 2.6 mm for the non-pregnant; these distinctions were viewed as clinically significant. Top expansions in measurement were shown during the powerful part of the development, as opposed to the last resting position. Results from our computational reproduction propose that maternal joint stacking in an upstanding birthing position, like crouching, could open the power source of the birth trench and dynamic exercises might produce more prominent pelvic versatility than the similar static stance.

EFFECTS OF SQUAT ON THE PELVIS

The manner by which we move, the scope of movement we approach at our joints, and the limit with respect to us to stack the body inside and remotely, are subject to our capacity to relax.

While "relaxing" and "breathing activities" might be a popular expression inside the business of wellbeing, wellness and execution, I'm certain we can all appreciate, breathing isn't something new or novel.

We inhale as many as 20,000 times each day, and with every breath that we take, there are related developments inside the body that happen to empower us to move and adjust our body shape to finish the respiratory pattern of inward breath and exhalation. Each bone, muscle, tendon, ligament, organ, fascial compartment, etc, are completely impacted by breath.

The capacity for us to get to and keep up with the full respiratory cycle and its related developments, moving between the full outing of exhalation and inward breath, confoundingly affects our ability to travel through scopes of movements at the joints of our body.

In the present knowledge I need to take a gander at this, comparable to two of the most straightforward rec center staple activities, the Squat and the Deadlift, and utilize the Pelvis and Sacrum as models for the general movements that happen.

Consider all along nonetheless, that overall movements likewise happen through the foot, lower leg, lower appendage, ribcage, shoulder support, upper appendage and hand comparable to breath. However the case of the pelvis will ideally give the most visual portrayal.

We will zero in simply on the mechanics at the pelvis that empower us to accomplish these two development designs from the back to front. For this situation we're talking developments related with the pelvis, sacrum and pelvic floor as it connects with breath while crouching, pivoting and relaxing.

Ideally it will begin to give some knowledge into where people might battle with regards to getting to the scope of movement required, or why issues might emerge in execution under load.

In the event that we take a gander at the picture underneath, this is an extremely distorted illustration of the essential pelvic and thoracic stomach development related with inward breath and exhalation. You'll perceive how as we breathe in, the thoracic stomach plummets and pushes downwards into our stomach cavity, the descending draw of the thoracic stomach makes a vacuum of negative tension that permits the lungs above to grow and fill.

All the while, this makes the pelvic stomach plunge to catch the descending development of the organs and viscera into the stomach hole.

On exhalation we see an inversion of these activities. The pelvic stomach agrees to push back facing the stomach contents as the thoracic stomach reascends into its more domed resting position.

UNDER NON-COMPENSATORY RESPIRATORY MECHANICS, THE Activities OF THE PELVIC AND THORACIC Stomach MIRROR One another. DESCENSION ON Inward breath, Rising ON EXHALATION.

To make it all the more likely to comprehend the impact of breath and relative movements of the pelvis on how we move, start to consider the pelvis in four fragments, a foremost (front) and back (back) split into left and right sides, for example, in the picture beneath. As we investigate the two developments today, and more perplexing developments as we go on with future posts, this will help a ton in laying out where development is happening inside the pelvis.

In the following chart underneath we have the development of the pelvis during inward breath. While the bolts might address a more extensive scope of movement change that would normally be related with a mollusk breath in, the development happening continues as before.

As we take in and the two stomachs slide, the pelvis needs to adjust shape to empower the tension being applied from above to have space for the stomach items to move into.

This is accomplished by an outside revolution of the ilium bones of the pelvis which opens the delta to empower the guts and viscera to move descending. As the gulf opens, the power source closes which empowers the muscular build of the pelvic floor to slide and "catch" the stomach contents. Similarly as a water balloon loaded up with water extends when held upstanding as the water pulls down on the balloon.

This adjustment of the place of the ilium bones into outer revolution, likewise changes the place of the hip attachments themselves into a more retroverted position in which they face all the more horizontally. This expands the outer turn limits of the hip joints themselves. The capacity for you to remotely pivot your hip is reliant upon your capacity to make this inward breath position of the two comparing stomachs, thoracic and pelvic and the related relative movements at the ilium and hip attachment.

Close by the development of the ilium and retroverted shape change of the hip attachments, we likewise see an adjustment of the place of the sacrum. Consider the sacrum a rudder that coordinates the development of the stomach hole inside the pelvis forward (anteriorly) and in reverse (posteriorly).

On inward breath, we see counter-nutation of the sacrum in which the sacrum slants in reverse to expand the opening and accessible space inside the pelvic gulf.

The blend of these three relative developments, outside pivot of the ilium, retroversion of the hip attachment and sacral counternutation, make our idea of a breathed ready of the pelvis.

In the event that we investigate the picture underneath in which we are gazing straight down inside the actual pelvis, we can perceive how this place of the pelvis makes development and flighty muscle movement in the foremost part both right and left, while making more pressure and concentric muscle action in the back piece of the pelvic floor.

We travel through the course of development. For this situation, the front extension of the pelvic floor is coordinating development downwards.

This is a basic prerequisite for our capacity to crouch down through full reach. Without these general movements happening, what might appear to be as a successful squat simply structure a visual point of view, may include compensatory developments to happen to accomplish a development without keeping up with this full outing of breath and the related developments.

On exhalation, we see an inversion of these three developments and the ilium, hip attachment and sacrum. The moves into the inside pivot, with the pelvic outlet opening to empower the pelvic floor to contract and reascend. We likewise see nutation of the sacrum, in which the base presently slants advances, and risk variant of the hip attachment which increments accessible inward turn of the hip joints themselves.

These overall developments see the sacrum, going about as a rudder, divert the tensions inside the pelvis. With the front pelvic stomach now more compressive and concentric and the back pelvic stomach more unusual and broad.

An individual ready to finish this full trip of breath with all general movements under wraps, should hence inside the pelvis approach ~60 levels of outer pivot and ~40 of inner revolution for a full journey all out of ~100 degrees.

To give a fast survey before we hop into the Squat and Deadlift, the breathed ready of the pelvis is one that is more;

Remotely pivoted at the ilium
Retroverted at the hip attachment
Counter-nutated at the sacrum
Extended in the front part of the pelvic floor
(coordinating development downwards)
Compacted in the back part of the pelvic floor
While the breathed out position of the pelvis is one that is more;

Inward pivoted at the ilium
Anteverted at the hip attachment
Nutated at the sacrum
Compacted in the front piece of the pelvic floor

Extended in the back part of the pelvic floor
(coordinating development in reverse)
Applying this into the developments of the Squat and
Deadlift essentially expects us to comprehend the
overall movements that happen as we travel through the
scope of every one of the two developments.

Starting with the Squat, we first need to see the value in
what gravity means for breath inside our resting stance
in standing.

Accepting we are stopping on two feet close to one
another, this addresses an inward breath position of the
pelvis with the overall movements at play. This is on the
grounds that we are constantly one-sided marginally
towards inward breath. We see this physiologically with
the idea of leftover lung volume. Indeed, even with our
fullest maximal deliberate exhalation, we actually have
some degree of air still inside our lungs to keep up with
the tensions we want inside to stay upstanding against
gravity.

WE HAVE Predisposition TOWARDS Inward breath
AND Outer Pivot AND Foster OUR Inner Turn Limits
Over the long run.

Any development subsequently starts with a respective
(two feet), even position, starting from our breath in
one-sided pelvic position.

As we slide through the Squat, we move from inward breath (~0-60 degrees) to exhalation (~60-120 degrees), and back to inward breath (~120-160 degrees) in the exceptionally base scope of the development. To effectively plummet into the Squat while keeping up with relative movement, we hence need to move between…

outer turn - inward pivot - outside revolution of the ilium on a proper femur
retroversion - risk rendition - retroversion of the hip attachments on a decent femur
counternutation - nutation and counternutation of the sacrum
These developments direct the inward tensions to grow adequately in the fitting regions to accomplish the profundity of the respectable.

On the re-rising of the Squat, we again see an inversion of these developments, starting from the base in a predisposition towards outer turn, retroversion and counter-nutation and traveling through inward pivot, bet variant and sacral nutation around the 90 degree point and back to more inward breath inclination, as we return to standing.

This center period of the development, the more inner turn one-sided, mid-range segment, is significant in our ability to control the plunge and produce force in the climb of the Squat.

In the event that we envision for instance, the contrast between crouching to resemble/90 levels of hip flexion, we might have the option to perceive how this includes development between inward breath to start, into exhalation around the 90 degree point, and a re-visitation of inward breath on standing. We can probably accomplish a Squat to 90 with just the capacity to accomplish the breathed out position of the pelvis from our beginning predisposition towards inward breath expecting relative movements are set up.

Nonetheless, in accomplishing full profundity and advancement the mid reaches (60-120 degrees), we really want full relative movements of inward breath and exhalation to happen. We want inward breath to exhalation and a re-visitation of inward breath to catch the full profundity required.

So to outline, our Squat example expects us to direct and control powers straightforwardly down into the pelvis.

To accomplish full profundity in a Squat in which our sitting bones are over our heels, we really want to the pelvis to accomplish its full scope of relative movements of inward breath and exhalation as it connects with outside and inner pivot, hip attachment retroversion and bet form, as well as sacral counternutation and nutation, among a large group of other relative movements inside the body that we will examine in ongoing bits of knowledge.

Once more moving onto our Deadlift model, we require the body to move between its breathed out and breathed in places. In any case, the degree in which we accomplish these overall movements changes.

From a respective, balanced position with a pelvis more one-sided towards outside turn, retroversion, sacral counternutation and a whimsically orientated extended front pelvic floor, we really want to divert inside strain to make a pivot movement, instead of a hunching down activity.

To accomplish this, we want to posteriorly make pressure in the foremost piece of the pelvic floor and develop. This diverts the stomach contents out of the shadow space we've made, empowering a pivot activity where the hips move posteriorly (back) as opposed to poorly (down).

As we ought to now be starting to get a handle on, this back development is the breathed out position of the pelvis with the general movements of inward revolution, risk form of the hip attachments (expanding femur interior turn), and sacral nutation.

Breathe in - Breathe out - Breathe in

We will have all seen people who can drop into a Squat with apparently practically zero obstruction yet battle in developments that include pivoting like a Deadlift,

Romanian Deadlift or Single Leg Deadlift. They come up short on ability to accomplish this breathed out position of the pelvis to make force into the ground.

Moreover we will have seen people who are serious areas of strength for unimaginably pivoting developments like the Deadlift, however basically can't under 90 degrees inside a Squat without a few extremely clear, clear pay. They miss the mark on ability to accomplish the breath ready of the pelvis to make extension and profundity inside a Squat.

The capacity to accomplish these general movements is subject to our capacity to keep up with the full journey of breath inward breath to exhalation and back once more.

However while we might comprehend these movements comparable to how we ought to move and breathe under ideal circumstances with practically no imperatives, people are intricate.

We have hereditary variables that will incline us more towards inward breath or exhalation, we have shallow systems created through preparing and way of life decisions that can again modify these general movements and the full trip of relaxing.

Yet, essentially, we can't separate these two elements, moving is endlessly breathing.

CHAPTER 4

FOCUSING ON THE DEAL(BIRTHING)

1. Enable yourself
Each lady is unique. Our bodies are unique, our children are unique and no 2 births are something very similar.

That is the reason figuring out more about work and birth is helpful. Seeing more about your choices, and the upsides and downsides of each, can assist you with feeling more sure about arriving at conclusions about how you need to convey your child.

You can likewise converse with your birthing specialist assuming that there is anything you're especially worried about. They will respond to any inquiries you have and make sense of how to convey your child securely in each conceivable situation.

You may likewise find antenatal classes supportive. Ask your birthing specialist, wellbeing guest or GP about NHS classes locally, or find a Public Labor Trust (NCT) course close to you.

NHS antenatal classes are free however the NCT might charge an expense. It's fine to go to more than 1 kind of class assuming you need to. You may likewise have the option to view the birthing offices at your clinic. This might assist you with choosing where you need to conceive an offspring and picture how things might be on the day.

"I went in feeling pretty pre-arranged the initial time. I watched a great deal of birth recordings, read books, did dynamic birth courses and explored situating works out. I was fortunate that my most memorable birth was perfect. The second time I was bricking it! I was stressed about the way that I'd adapt assuming it went distinctively to what I knew. So I went through my old notes with my birthing specialist and I did more research through the Relationship for Upgrades in Maternity Administrations (Points). I encourage mums to do their own examination on anything they are stressed over. Engage yourself with information so you feel like you can pursue your own choices."

2. Set up your brain
Make an effort not to pay attention to harrowing tales about work as these are truly pointless on the off chance that you're feeling apprehensive. Attempt to recall that for each terrible experience, there is a mum out there with a positive story to tell.

This can be hard, particularly in the event that you've had a terrible encounter yourself. In any case, attempt to think decidedly however much as could be expected.

Loads of mums let us know it truly assists with having an uplifting perspective.

"Something that truly decreased my apprehension was hearing positive birth accounts. I searched out the "I sniffled and my child was conceived" type stories, which caused me to accept that having a work with negligible intervention was conceivable."

"My companion expressed that subsequent to hearing my introduction to the world story, she was so empowered she traversed the majority of her own work at home easily. I surmise a ton of the time it's tied in with accepting that you can make it happen."

"I found conversing with my companions who had conceived an offspring about their encounters truly accommodating. It truly quieted my nerves."

"I looked into positive birth stories on the web and read positive books, which I think affected my positive perspective."

3. Set up your body
Work frequently requires strength and endurance, so setting up your body for it is significant. Practice during pregnancy can likewise be an incredible way to de-stress.

You could give finding a shot about antenatal activity classes close to you. For instance, a pregnancy yoga class can be truly useful. It will assist you with setting your child up in a decent way for birth, train you in positions to help you through work, and give a few unwinding and breathing procedures to assist you with keeping cool-headed. However, any kind of activity is great. In the event that you don't have the opportunity or cash to join a class, only taking a stroll in the park will be useful.

"My most memorable child was brought into the world consecutively with forceps. I needed to keep away from this reoccurring. I went to a functioning birth studio where I found out about getting the child into a decent position, how my pelvis shape could impact work and rehearsed activities to help me through it. As anticipated, my subsequent work slowed down at a similar point as the first yet, rather than overreacting, I had the option to attempt various positions. I felt more in charge and my subsequent child was brought into the world with practically no clinical help."

Figure out more about practice in pregnancy.

4. Practice unwinding strategies
Utilizing breathing strategies can assist with quieting your nerves (when working) and control the aggravation. You can rehearse the entire way through pregnancy to guarantee you're open to utilizing them when work begins.

"Gain proficiency with a few unwinding and breathing strategies. I didn't do a hypnobirthing course, yet I purchased a book and Disc and it helped tremendously with a long and unsavory enlistment. Regardless of it finishing in a crisis c-area, I felt I'd had the most ideal work insight up to that point, the situation being what it is."

Reflection and representation can assist you with loosening up through pregnancy and during work. Regardless of whether your work goes the manner in which you arranged you might in any case have the option to utilize the procedures you've learned.

"The best thing I did was contemplation, including positive perception. After a troublesome first birth I found I could make my own positive space and energy the subsequent time. I felt quiet and together in any event, when I was in torment."

Correlative treatments, for example, needle therapy may likewise assist you with unwinding. Simply ensure your acupuncturist is completely qualified and that they utilize dispensable needles at each treatment meeting. Let your specialist know that you're pregnant as well, in light of the fact that specific needle therapy can't be utilized securely in pregnancy.

"I was frantic to stay away from enlistment with number 2. I was really worried towards the finish of my pregnancy, so I chose to attempt needle therapy. The acupuncturist significantly altered my perspective and, little by little, I began to relax. Work got going normally and I genuinely accept it was an outlook thing and that I expected to unwind and zero in on a tad. A great deal of these treatments, regardless of whether they work, do assist you with unwinding, which is essential to get the right chemicals streaming."

A few mums have found hypnobirthing valuable.

"Since I blacked out during a school science example watching a lady in labor, I've been totally scared of conceiving an offspring. At the point when I fell pregnant I realized I needed to assume command and do something positive to help me through the following 9 months. I chose to do an escalated hypnobirthing course. It was expensive yet worth each penny as from that second on I felt substantially more in charge. The positive confirmations, genuine encounters, book, Cd and work on hypnobirthing meetings had the universe of effect in the development. I paid attention to the Compact disc (and digital recordings I downloaded) consistently as a general rule for quite some time. I'd as a rule nod off before the end. Toward the finish of my pregnancy I was loose and blissful, and not especially worried about conceiving an offspring by any means! The hypnobirthing helped me for the initial 12 hours of work. I wasn't terrified and felt a genuine feeling of quiet."

5. Contemplate your introduction to the world arrangement
A birth plan can be a helpful approach to imparting every one of your desires, concerns and decisions rapidly and successfully, especially when you move to dynamic work and probably shouldn't (or have the option to) have significant conversations with your maternity specialist, or on the other hand in the event that there's a staff change. Simply recall that work doesn't generally go to anticipate the day, so you might need to be somewhat adaptable.

"After a horrendous first birth, I was encouraged to utilize my introduction to the world to convey my tensions to clinical staff. I recorded what turned out badly the first time, and how I needed to be dealt with distinctively this time. It implied I didn't need to continue onward over my most memorable birth story and all the staff were completely mindful of my circumstance and wants (for instance I needed to abstain from having an epidural, having endured the epidural cerebral pain for the first time). They comprehended that I battled with absence of correspondence for the first time, so ensured this wasn't an issue. In correlation, my subsequent work was significantly more loose and I felt more upheld and in charge."

Second time mums
In the event that you're worried about conceiving an offspring once more, it could assist with discussing what happened the first time round.

Interviewing administration
Most emergency clinics have help for mums who might want to discuss their experience conceiving an offspring. It may very well be known as a birth reflection or birth untimely ideas administration. Going over your introduction to the world involvement in a maternity specialist - but lengthy after you conceived an offspring - can assist you with figuring out what occurred and maybe assist you with adapting to any tensions about doing it once more.

Figure out more about feelings of dread toward labor.

Go over your work notes
Talk through your work notes exhaustively with a clinical expert, similar to your maternity specialist. This will assist you with filling in any holes in your memory, ask inquiries regarding for what valid reason things happened, the manner in which they did and allow you an opportunity to figure out what you might want to do any other way. Figure out how you can get to your notes.

* 9 7 9 8 3 6 6 6 8 4 8 5 9 *